DEMENTIA, ALZHEIMER'S DISEASE STAGES, TREATMENTS, AND OTHER MEDICAL CONSIDERATIONS

Laura Town and Karen Kassel

Silver Hills Press
Zionsville, IN 46077

ISBN: 978-1-943414-07-9

Production Credits:
Authors: Laura Town and Karen Kassel
Publisher: Silver Hills Press
Photos: All images used under license from Shutterstock.com

Social Media Connections:
Laura Town
Twitter: @laurawtown
LinkedIn: http://www.linkedin.com/in/lauratown
GooglePlus: http://plus.google.com/u/0/117415714202281042310/posts
Pinterest: http://www.pinterest.com/laurat0428

Karen Kassel
Twitter: @KarenKassel1
LinkedIn: http://www.linkedin.com/pub/karen-kassel/62/2b/915/

TABLE OF CONTENTS

DEMENTIA, ALZHEIMER'S DISEASE STAGES, TREATMENTS, AND OTHER MEDICAL CONSIDERATIONS

Approximately 35 million individuals worldwide have Alzheimer's disease, with 5.2 million Americans being treated for the condition. These estimates are expected to triple by 2050 if no means of curing or preventing Alzheimer's disease is discovered. Alzheimer's disease primarily affects individuals age 65 and older, with more than 96% of reported U.S. cases occurring in this population. The likelihood of developing Alzheimer's disease increases with age, as individuals over the age of 85 have a 50% chance of developing the disease; however, symptoms associated with Alzheimer's disease are not simply a normal part of the aging process. Rather, because age is a major risk factor for Alzheimer's disease, more cases of Alzheimer's disease will emerge as individuals begin to live longer.

Alzheimer's disease was first discovered in 1906 by Dr. Alois Alzheimer, who encountered a woman with an odd mental illness. Her symptoms included memory loss, odd behaviors, and difficulties with language. After the woman's death, Dr. Alzheimer examined her brain and found abnormal changes, including what are now called plaques and tangles. The disease was named after the doctor who first noted its characteristics, and it has increased in prevalence ever since. In 2014, Alzheimer's disease was noted as the sixth-leading cause of death in the United States.

Medical Description

Alzheimer's disease causes the deterioration and death of nerve cells—called neurons—in the brain. A neuron's basic role is to transmit information, both to other neurons and to other parts of the body. Neurons accomplish this task by producing chemical and electrical signals that carry bursts of information from one place to another. Together, neurons form the nervous system, which is fundamental to an individual's ability to translate thoughts into words and actions. When neurons die, the communication between neurons and the body break down. For individuals with Alzheimer's disease, this neuronal death causes personality changes and a decline in their ability to remember and think coherently.

The death of neurons in different parts of the brain affects different areas of functioning. In Alzheimer's disease, the destruction of neurons in the hippocampus, located in the middle of the base of the brain, causes failures in short-term memory, whereas neuron death in the cerebral cortex, which is the largest part of the brain

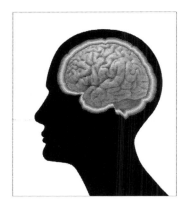 that is covered in the iconic folds, affects the ability to think, plan, and form correct judgments. The symptoms of Alzheimer's disease begin gradually, but as time progresses and more brain cells die, the memory loss, confusion, and personality changes begin to be more severe. Ultimately, brain cell death progresses until the individual is no longer able to function independently or communicate coherently, eventually leading to death.

Dementia

Dementia and Alzheimer's disease are often treated as interchangeable terms. However, dementia is a generic term used to describe a group of symptoms, whereas Alzheimer's disease is one specific type of dementia. *Dementia* refers to a decline in mental acuity so severe that it begins to impact an individual's daily functioning. Researchers believe 60–80% of all dementia cases are related to Alzheimer's disease and the remaining 20–40% of cases are related to a variety of other types of dementia. The following checklist highlights some of the main characteristics of dementia.

Checklist: Characteristics of dementia

☐ Impaired thinking

☐ Impaired judgment and reasoning

☐ Impaired memory, especially short-term memory

☐ Reduction in ability to perform everyday activities

☐ Difficulty communicating normally

☐ Periods of confusion

☐ Decreased focus

- [ ] Inability to pay attention to tasks

- [ ] Difficulty with visual perceptions

- [ ] Visual hallucinations

In most cases of dementia, symptoms begin slowly and progress over time. However, in some situations, usually those involving dementia-like symptoms brought on by medications, symptoms can appear very quickly. The symptoms of dementia vary considerably from individual to individual, but all cases of dementia involve impairment to core mental functions in at least two of five major areas: memory, communication and language, ability to focus and pay attention, ability to reason and form judgments, and visual perception. High-functioning, highly intelligent individuals can often devise clever compensating mechanisms that enable them to hide these symptoms for a long time, which makes it more difficult to detect, and thus treat, their dementia. My (Laura's) father, for example, was a professor, and when he would use strange or complex words to describe something simple, no one would find it odd. He was also getting older, so we did not question his decision to hire someone to mow his lawn or his decision to eat out at every meal, but in reality he no longer knew how to start the lawn mower or use the microwave.

Because dementia is often progressive, you should seek diagnosis and treatment for a loved one as early as possible if you notice that they are having difficulty in one of the five core areas of mental function. Early diagnosis and treatment is essential to delaying the progression of Alzheimer's disease.

Classic Alzheimer's Disease

Most cases of Alzheimer's disease appear when an individual is 65 years old or older. However, changes occur in the brain even before symptoms appear. Proteins called beta-amyloid begin depositing in the brain before an individual experiences memory loss. As these proteins are deposited, they form amyloid *plaques*, which are clumps of amyloid protein pieces that are stuck together in an unusable form. In addition, the disorganization of tau proteins in nerve cells prevents normal transport of nutrients, eventually resulting in nerve death. This disorganization of tau proteins lead to *tangles*. Together, plaques and tangles are the distinguishing pathological brain features of Alzheimer's disease. However, these plaques and tangles cannot be seen with modern brain imaging devices and can only be identified upon autopsy after an individual has passed away. This makes diagnosing Alzheimer's disease more complicated.

Two common views regarding plaques and tangles are in opposition to each other. The most common view is that plaques and tangles are pathogenic, contributing to the progression of Alzheimer's disease. As plaques build up, nerve cells are less able to communicate effectively with one another, slowing cognitive processing within the brain. These damaged nerve cells begin to die, forming tangles from twisted strands of tau protein. This nerve damage then contributes to the symptoms of Alzheimer's disease. In contrast, a view that is gaining favor is that the formation of plaques and tangles is actually a protective antioxidant mechanism used by the brain in response to stress on the nerve cells. In this view, the true underlying cause of the stress and symptoms is still unknown. Regardless of the view about the role of plaques and tangles in Alzheimer's disease, scientists agree that Alzheimer's disease involves the breakdown of nerve cells and neural functioning in the brain.

Risk Factors

Alzheimer's disease is a progressive disease that worsens over time. The cause of Alzheimer's disease is not yet understood. A combination of genetic, environmental, and lifestyle factors working together over time can cause Alzheimer's disease to develop, but each of these factors can vary in the importance of the role it plays depending on the individual. Many people who develop Alzheimer's disease begin to experience symptoms later in life, generally in their 60s and 70s, which eventually leads to diagnosis. Women have a greater risk of developing Alzheimer's disease than men, most likely because women tend to live longer. Alzheimer's disease is not a normal part of aging, but it is becoming more prevalent as the population ages. Some common risk factors for Alzheimer's disease are described in the following checklist.

Checklist: Risk factors for Alzheimer's disease

- ☐ **Age.** The leading risk factor for Alzheimer's disease is age. Once an individual reaches 65, the likelihood of developing the disease increases substantially. By age 85, the risk becomes close to 50%. In fact, people who are 85 or older have the highest risk of developing Alzheimer's disease out of any other population.

☐ **Genetics.** Alzheimer's disease tends to run in families, especially in early-onset cases, which occur when the disease appears in individuals younger than age 65. Understanding your family's genetic history of Alzheimer's disease will help you prepare for future medical problems. If a first-order family member (e.g., parent or sibling) has the disease, you are likely more susceptible. If a second-order family member (e.g., grandparent, aunt, uncle, half sibling) has the disease, you may also be more susceptible to Alzheimer's disease.

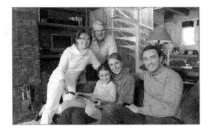

☐ **Diet and exercise.** Infrequent exercise and an unhealthy diet are both considered risk factors for developing Alzheimer's disease. This is due to an imbalance or deficiency of nutrients consistent with an unhealthy diet as well as the extra strain put on the body (particularly the heart) when a person does not exercise regularly.

☐ **Smoking.** Individuals who smoke are at higher risk for having a stroke, having a heart attack, and developing high cholesterol and blood pressure. All of these factors increase a person's risk of developing Alzheimer's disease later in life.

☐ **Alcohol.** Chronic (i.e., long-term) and heavy alcohol use has been shown to increase the risk of developing dementia. The correlation between heavy drinking and Alzheimer's disease is difficult to study, as alcoholic dementia and Alzheimer's disease present many of the same symptoms.

☐ **Uncontrolled chronic diseases.** Uncontrolled diseases (i.e., diseases that are not adequately controlled through medical treatment) such as diabetes, high cholesterol, and high blood pressure can increase the risk of developing Alzheimer's disease.

☐ **Lifestyle choices.** Individuals who choose to participate in high-impact sports (e.g., football) or other risky behaviors increase their likelihood of decreased cognitive functioning as time progresses. This is due to their elevated risk of frequent head injuries, which substantially increase their chances of developing dementia.

☐ **Chemical exposure.** A link exists between exposure to the pesticide DDT (dichlorodiphenyltrichloroethane) and development of late-onset Alzheimer's disease. This pesticide has been outlawed in the United States since 1972, but many other countries around the world still use it. Thus, imported fruits, vegetables, and fish could potentially contain high amounts of DDT.

☐ **Chronic high stress.** Individuals with frequent high stress are at an increased risk for developing various forms of dementia. Similarly, individuals who experience stress while suffering from Alzheimer's disease often notice an acceleration in the progression of their symptoms.

☐ **Depression.** Chronic depression is a risk factor for many diseases, including heart disease and Alzheimer's disease.

Prevention

Research has yet to identify any actions individuals can take to prevent the development of Alzheimer's disease. However, many methods that could delay the development and slow the progression of the disease have been suggested. Some of these methods include changes to exercise, diet, and lifestyle habits, as suggested by the risk factors for Alzheimer's disease. These changes are often recommended

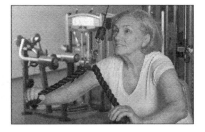

because they promote healthy brain activity and mental acuity. The healthier and more active an individual's brain is, the lower the risk for memory problems. The following checklist highlights some such changes that can help promote brain health.

Checklist: Slowing the progression of Alzheimer's disease

Diet:

☐ Include brain-healthy foods in your diet, such as fish, nuts, dark leafy greens, berries, fruits, avocadoes, and eggs.

☐ Increase your intake of foods rich in vitamin E, such as nuts, whole grains, dark greens, and vegetable oils.

- ☐ Employ the Mediterranean diet, which consists of fish, fruits, vegetables, olive oil, and red wines. This diet primarily avoids red meat and saturated fats.

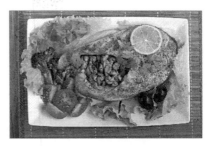

- ☐ Increase your intake of meals high in vitamin B12 and folate, including non-fatty meats (i.e., non-fried, non-breaded meats that are naturally low in fat or have the fat removed), fish, eggs, cheese, beans, whole grains, and green vegetables.

- ☐ Avoid the saturated fatty acids found in fatty meats, butter, fried foods, and baked goods.

Exercise:

- ☐ Develop a regular exercise regimen. Exercise should include 30 to 60 minutes of aerobic activity (e.g., walking, running, swimming, biking) three to five times each week. However, you or your loved one will benefit from any amount of exercise, even if it is only light exercise two or three times per week. Water activities such as swimming or water aerobics are recommended for individuals with joint problems.

- ☐ Engage in resistance training (strengthening the muscles) at least once a week up to two to three times per week. Studies have shown that resistance training in older adults increases mental acuity.

- ☐ Stay active as often as possible, avoiding a high percentage of sedentary activities such as watching television.

- ☐ Consult with a physician before beginning an exercise regimen, especially if you or your loved one have any health conditions that would prevent strenuous activity, such as heart or lung disease or extreme obesity.

Lifestyle:

- ☐ Avoid smoking tobacco products.

- ☐ Avoid heavy drinking and controlled substances not prescribed by a doctor.

- ☐ Take steps to manage your blood pressure.

- ☐ Monitor and regulate your blood sugar levels, if you have diabetes.

- ☐ Watch your cholesterol levels and eat foods shown to lower cholesterol such as oatmeal, high fiber foods, fish, nuts, olive oil, soy, fruits, beans, eggplant, okra, and whole grains. Coincidentally, these foods are also recommended for improving brain health.

- ☐ Work to maintain a healthy body weight.

- ☐ Engage in activities that keep your mind active, such as reading, writing, doing puzzles, working on crossword puzzles, watching plays, gardening, quilting, knitting, and learning new things.

Warning Signs

If your loved one has any of the risk factors for Alzheimer's disease, you should watch them for early symptoms, especially if your loved one is age 60 or older. Symptoms that indicate Alzheimer's disease include actions or changes that cannot be explained by the normal aging process. The following checklist discusses some common warning signs that occur.

Checklist: Warning signs

- ☐ Your loved one has been experiencing memory loss that impacts their daily life, such as forgetting dates and events and having difficulty remembering recently learned facts.

- ☐ Your loved one frequently repeats stories or questions, even if they have told the story or asked the question multiple times in the past few minutes.

- ☐ Your loved one is experiencing problems concentrating.

- ☐ Your loved one has become confused about who they are.

- ☐ Your loved one's appearance or attention to personal hygiene has changed.

- ☐ Your loved one finds it difficult to complete routine tasks at home.

- ☐ Your loved one takes longer than usual to complete regular tasks.

- ☐ Your loved one begins to misplace things more frequently.

- [ ] Your loved one finds it difficult to organize and keep track of their bills every month.

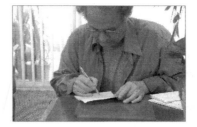

- [ ] Your loved one has forgotten to pay some of their bills.

- [ ] Your loved one forgets the steps in processes they are accustomed to performing (e.g., forgetting how to play a once-favored game).

- [ ] Your loved one has stopped participating in a once-favored hobby.

- [ ] Your loved one has become disoriented and forgotten how they arrived at a particular location.

- [ ] Your loved one appears confused during conversations, as if they are having difficulty following what is being said.

- [ ] Your loved one experiences difficulties while speaking, including forgetting words, repeating ideas, or not being able to finish their thoughts.

- [ ] Your loved one has stopped socializing with friends.

- [ ] Your loved one has more frequent vision problems, including difficulties reading and seeing clearly while driving.

- [ ] Your loved one has changes in personality and/or moods that were not previously common.

- [ ] Your loved one has started to demonstrate extreme emotions, such as anger and sadness, on a more regular basis.

If your loved one displays any of the warning signs of Alzheimer's disease, encourage them to make an appointment with a physician to determine if they have Alzheimer's disease or another common form of dementia.

Choosing a Doctor

Helping your loved one choose a doctor, or choosing one for them, can be a very difficult task. Your loved one's primary care physician will probably not be the only doctor your loved one will need. They will also likely need to see a neurologist or another specialist with extensive experience treating individuals with Alzheimer's disease. You will need to find a doctor in whom you and your loved one are confident will provide the best care. This will help create trust between you, your loved one, and your doctor, relieving some of the stress associated with Alzheimer's disease. The following checklist highlights some questions to consider when choosing a doctor for Alzheimer's care.

Checklist: Questions to consider when choosing a doctor

☐ Does the doctor specialize in Alzheimer's care? If so, for how many years?

☐ Does the doctor accept your loved one's insurance?

☐ Does the doctor come recommended by others (e.g., primary care physician or other medical professional, or patients or family members of patients)?

☐ What is the doctor's reputation in the community? Have you heard any negative criticism about the doctor?

☐ Is the doctor's office within a reasonable drive from your loved one's home?

☐ Is the staff friendly when you or your loved one call to make an appointment?

☐ Is the doctor's office convenient for your loved one to reach? Are close parking spots available, and is the office easy to find and access?

☐ Does the doctor have reduced wait times? Lengthy wait times can be difficult for individuals with Alzheimer's disease.

☐ Does the doctor complete a full medical history during the first visit?

☐ Does the doctor conduct any tests during the first visit to determine the cause and severity of your loved one's memory loss?

☐ Is the doctor planning to rule out all other possible causes of your loved one's symptoms? What tests will the doctor use to rule out these symptoms? Will these tests be covered by insurance?

☐ Do you and your loved one agree with the tests the doctor plans to run during future appointments?

- ☐ Does the doctor take time to listen to your concerns and answer all of your questions?

- ☐ Do you or your loved one feel rushed during the appointment?

- ☐ Does the doctor explain things clearly?

- ☐ Is the doctor friendly and professional?

- ☐ Does your loved one like the doctor?

- ☐ Has the doctor done or said anything to make you or your loved one uncomfortable?

- ☐ Is the doctor willing to outline a personal plan of care if your loved one does have Alzheimer's disease?

- ☐ Do you and your loved one agree with the plan of care proposed by the doctor?

- ☐ Does the doctor support the treatment methods your loved one prefers (e.g., if your loved one wants to use alternative or natural treatments)? Is the doctor familiar with these treatments?

- ☐ Is the doctor willing to continue treating your loved one at a long-term care facility if your loved one is unable to travel to the doctor's office?

- ☐ Does the doctor, or his office, have an ongoing relationship with trusted geriatric and psychiatric medical professionals in the area?

Some individuals go to their family physician or primary care physician if they suspect they have Alzheimer's disease. Although this may seem like a logical choice, some experts in the field believe this decision could lead to a misdiagnosis. If your loved one has been going to the same physician for many years, the doctor's extensive knowledge of your loved one's medical history could affect their ability to correctly diagnose your loved one. In addition, your loved one's primary care physician may not be experienced in diagnosing and treating Alzheimer's disease. Your loved one's primary doctor, however, could be a great resource for a referral to a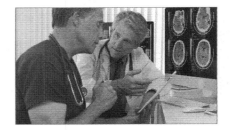

doctor who specializes in Alzheimer's disease. Several types of doctors specialize in treating and diagnosing neurological diseases or diseases common to older patients, including Alzheimer's disease. The following checklist describes these different types of doctors.

Checklist: Doctors who treat Alzheimer's disease

- ☐ **Geriatrician.** This type of doctor specializes in the care of older adults. They are able to diagnose Alzheimer's disease, and due to their specialization probably see the disease often. Geriatricians are trained to see how an illness is affecting their patient physically, socially, and emotionally.

- ☐ **Neurologist.** Neurology deals with disorders that involve the nervous system, which includes the brain. Because the nervous system is so extensive, many neurologists specialize in particular areas. If the doctor specializes in neurodegenerative disorders, including Alzheimer's disease, then they will likely have a lot of experience diagnosing and treating Alzheimer's disease.

- ☐ **Psychiatrist and neuropsychiatrist.** Psychiatrists are doctors who specialize in disorders that affect the brain. They work to understand the relationship between emotional and physical illness. Geriatric psychiatrists focus particularly on those 65 and older who have psychological conditions. Neuropsychiatrists focus on the interrelation between neurological and psychological disorders, such as Alzheimer's disease.

- ☐ **Psychologist and neuropsychologist.** Psychologists help individuals deal with complex emotional difficulties, such as extreme anger, depression, and anxiety. They often use various forms of therapy to help their patients. Neuropsychologists are trained in the interrelationship of disorders of the brain and the resulting behaviors. These professionals are able to diagnose Alzheimer's disease.

Diagnosing Alzheimer's Disease

The earlier Alzheimer's disease is diagnosed, the earlier your loved one can start planning for their future. Alzheimer's disease is a progressive disease that can sometimes advance very quickly, so early detection can be extremely beneficial. The earlier treatment of the disease begins, the more time your loved one will likely have to spend with family, take care of legal matters (see *Advance Directives, Durable Power of Attorney, Wills, and Other Legal Considerations*), organize future living arrangements (see *Home Care, Long-Term Care, Memory Care Units, and Other Living Arrangements*), make their wishes known, and prepare for the future. If you suspect that your loved one has Alzheimer's disease or if your loved one has recently been diagnosed with Alzheimer's disease, you and your loved one should make a list of questions to ask the doctor. The following checklist highlights some questions you or your loved one should ask the doctor both before and after diagnosis.

Checklist: Questions to ask the doctor

Before diagnosis:

☐ How long does it take to diagnose Alzheimer's disease?

☐ What kinds of tests are involved?

☐ Will my loved one's insurance company cover all of these tests?

☐ Could there be other factors causing these symptoms?

☐ What will you do to rule out other potential problems that could be causing the symptoms?

☐ Is this amount of memory loss abnormal for my loved one's age range?

After diagnosis:

☐ How quickly does the disease usually progress?

☐ Will my loved one need to begin seeing a specialist? If so, is there anyone you can personally recommend?

☐ How long does it generally take to get an appointment with a specialist?

☐ What treatment options are available (e.g., medications, therapies)? Which would you recommend?

☐ What are the benefits and risks of treatment? What are the common side effects of medications used to treat Alzheimer's disease?

☐ Are there non-drug therapies that have shown success?

☐ Should I look into clinical trials for my loved one?

☐ Are there any clinical trials in particular that you would recommend?

☐ Will the symptoms of Alzheimer's disease interact with any other medical conditions my loved one has?

☐ Are there other medical or community resources you can recommend?

When your loved one goes to their doctor's appointment, the doctor will want to know the specifics about any symptoms your loved one is experiencing. If possible, you and your loved one should keep a list of symptoms to give the doctor, including the severity and frequency of each symptom and an example or two of what happened when each symptom occurred. You and your loved one should be completely honest about these symptoms and talk to the doctor about any concerns you are having. Once the doctor has a better idea of your loved one's symptoms, they can begin tests to rule out other ailments to determine whether your loved one does indeed have Alzheimer's disease. The following checklist details some of the tests conducted to diagnose Alzheimer's disease.

Checklist: Diagnostic tests

☐ A full medical history will be conducted to assess other potential reasons for the symptoms, such as drug interactions.

☐ A physical examination will be conducted to check for signs of other ailments, such as stroke or Parkinson's disease.

☐ Lab tests will be done to rule out vitamin deficiencies and thyroid problems.

☐ Psychological evaluations may be done to assess for signs of depression. Symptoms of depression and symptoms of Alzheimer's disease can be similar, and the presence of depression in someone with Alzheimer's disease may lead to faster progression of Alzheimer's disease and/or suicidal thoughts.

☐ Mental status tests will be performed to determine how much the cognitive impairment and memory loss has progressed. These may include being asked to remember a short list of words or do simple math problems.

☐ Tests such as the mini-mental state exam (MMSE) and the mini-cog will be conducted to evaluate thinking and memory skills. For example, your loved one may be given the name of three or four different objects and then asked to repeat them a few minutes later.

☐ A mini-mental state exam tests an individual's range of mental skills by asking several questions in a short period of time. Scores on the MMSE indicate whether a person has mild, moderate, or severe dementia: Out of a possible 30 points, 20–24 points suggests mild dementia, 13–20 points suggests moderate dementia, and fewer than 12 points suggests severe dementia.

☐ For the MMSE, most adults without dementia should be able to answer the exam questions correctly without trouble. For example, the exam asks test takers to orient themselves to time (year, season, date, day, month) and location (country, state, city, hospital, floor). The test taker might be shown a picture of a watch and asked to identify what they see or be asked to recall in order the names of three common nouns the test taker just heard, such as rope/duck/jar. Timing for answering the questions is often as short as ten seconds, but even so, the questions should be easy for anyone without the impairment of dementia to answer correctly.

☐ The mini-cog is a similar mental status test in two parts. In the first part, the test taker is told the names of three common objects that they must remember and be able to repeat several minutes later. This is similar to MMSE questions, except that in the mini-cog a few minutes elapse before the test taker must respond with the correct answer. The second part is to correctly draw a clock face with the numbers in the proper order and positions. The clock face must also show the hour and minute hands pointing to a specific time, such as two o'clock.

☐ No test is definitive, but mental status tests such as the MMSE and mini-cog are important diagnostic tools that can help a physician make a determination of dementia in a patient. The MMSE can also be used to chart the progress of dementia. A person with Alzheimer's disease will on average lose two to four points from their MMSE score with every passing year.

☐ CT scans may be done to rule out other ailments and identify the progression of the disease in the brain.

☐ An MRI may be done to show doctors a detailed image of the brain and rule out other potential diseases.

☐ Studies are ongoing regarding the use of a cerebrospinal fluid test for diagnosing Alzheimer's disease. In this test, cerebrospinal fluid is collected and tested for specific forms of beta-amyloid and tau proteins associated with plaques and tangles. However, this test is not yet standardized and is primarily used in research and clinical trials.

☐ PET scans are another newer technology being used to detect amyloid and other diagnostic markers in the brain. However, these scans are also primarily used in research and clinical trials until greater standardization is developed.

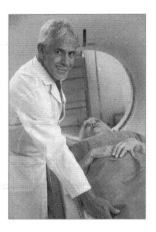

Some tests to diagnose Alzheimer's disease may be done on the first visit, but many of them will be conducted over the span of a few weeks. Remember that the only definitive, standardized test for Alzheimer's disease is a brain biopsy, which is not conducted until after death. Therefore, physicians must take your loved one through a series of tests to rule out other diseases and other forms of dementia before they can diagnose your loved one with Alzheimer's disease. Then, after all the testing, if your loved one is diagnosed with Alzheimer's disease, the doctor will likely give a diagnosis of "possible" or "probable" Alzheimer's disease, since no one test can conclusively diagnose Alzheimer's disease while your loved one is alive. Physicians experienced in diagnosing and treating Alzheimer's disease can usually diagnose Alzheimer's disease with 90% accuracy. Once additional biomarker tests such as the cerebrospinal fluid test and PET scans become more widely available, this percentage may increase.

Differential Diagnosis

When your loved one's doctor is going through the testing process to determine whether your loved one has Alzheimer's disease, they must rule out several other types of dementia before making the final diagnosis. Although Alzheimer's disease is the most common form of dementia, several other forms of dementia account for 20–40% of all dementia cases. Each form of dementia presents in different ways, with individualized symptoms and changes to the brain. The following checklist discusses the various forms of dementia.

Checklist: Different forms of dementia

☐ **Alzheimer's disease.** Alzheimer's disease is the most common form of dementia. It manifests with difficulties remembering events and people stored in short-term memory and eventually progresses to difficulties with long-term memory, such as not being able to remember one's parents and/or childhood. Later symptoms also include difficulty walking, communicating, and swallowing. Typical brain changes include the accumulation of plaques and tangles.

☐ **Vascular dementia.** Vascular dementia is the second most common form of dementia and usually presents in individuals who have had a stroke or other medical event causing damage to blood vessels or arteries, especially those in the brain. However, not every individual who has had a stroke will develop vascular dementia. The main symptoms of vascular dementia are impaired judgment and difficulty making decisions and planning.

☐ **Lewy body dementia.** Lewy body dementia is the third most common form of dementia. It results from protein deposits in areas of the brain responsible for thinking, memory, and movement. As Lewy body dementia progresses, mental abilities begin to slow. Additionally, Lewy body dementia causes visual hallucinations and rigid muscle movements.

☐ **Parkinson's disease dementia.** As the symptoms of Parkinson's disease become more advanced, dementia usually results. Parkinson's disease dementia often presents with difficulty moving as well as other symptoms similar to Lewy body dementia.

☐ **Frontotemporal dementia.** Frontotemporal dementia occurs when a brain disorder cause the frontal lobe (in the front of the brain) and/or temporal lobes (at the sides of the brain) to shrink. These changes often result in symptoms affecting personality, including emotional outbursts, apathy, inappropriate social behaviors, or even loss of the ability to communicate. This form of dementia generally occurs when individuals are in their early 60s.

☐ **Creutzfeldt-Jakob disease.** Creutzfeldt-Jakob disease (CJD) is a rare and fatal disease that often presents with symptoms of memory loss, behavior changes, and difficulties with coordination and vision. Individuals usually develop CJD after the age of 60, and 90% of individuals die within one year of diagnosis.

☐ **Normal pressure hydrocephalus.** Normal pressure hydrocephalus is caused by the abnormal buildup of cerebrospinal fluid in the brain. Common symptoms include memory loss, problems walking, and inability to control one's bladder. Unlike most forms of dementia, these symptoms can sometimes be reversed by inserting a shunt to drain the excess fluid.

If, after extensive testing, your loved one is diagnosed with possible or probable Alzheimer's disease, understanding the stages of Alzheimer's disease will help you know what to expect and how to prepare for the future.

Stages of Alzheimer's Disease

In the past, Alzheimer's disease was described using a seven-stage system:

☐ Stage 1: No impairment

☐ Stage 2: Very mild decline

☐ Stage 3: Mild decline

☐ Stage 4: Moderate decline

☐ Stage 5: Moderately severe decline

☐ Stage 6: Severe decline

☐ Stage 7: Very severe decline

Most resources on Alzheimer's disease now condense that system into just three stages: mild, moderate, and severe. Regardless of the stage system used, remember that no two Alzheimer's disease patients are the same, so different patients will experience the symptoms associated with each stage at different times in different orders, and they might not all experience the same symptoms. One patient might experience some moderate symptoms early on, while another might not experience some symptoms of moderate decline until after the disease has progressed to a severe state.

Individuals with Alzheimer's disease live an average of eight years with the disease, but this can range from four years to 20 years, depending on age at diagnosis, severity of the disease at diagnosis, effectiveness of drug and other therapies, the progression rate of the disease, and the presence of other health conditions. Regardless of when during this timeframe your loved one experiences each symptom, they will likely go through a period of decline that progresses from mild impairment to severe impairment. In this book, we'll focus on the simplified three-stage model of Alzheimer's disease—mild, moderate, and severe—to describe the symptoms and prognosis common to each stage.

Stage 1: Mild

If your loved one is in stage 1, they are considered to have mild Alzheimer's disease. During stage 1, your loved one will experience a decline in the ability to remember as well as a decline in other cognitive functions. Your loved one will likely be diagnosed with possible or probable Alzheimer's disease at this stage. However, diagnosing Alzheimer's disease at this stage is often complicated because physicians may be unsure whether your loved one's symptoms are due to Alzheimer's disease or whether they are a normal sign of aging. Also, at this early stage, some highly functioning people may be able to compensate for their symptoms well enough that those symptoms aren't readily apparent.

Use your knowledge of your loved one to your advantage. Look not only for the symptoms outlined here, but also compare the symptoms to your loved one's normal personality and behavior. Look for changes that are warning signs and definitely not typical for your loved one.

Checklist: Symptoms in stage 1

☐ Gradual progression of memory loss, especially short-term memory

☐ Trouble recalling recent events, such as newly learned information or recent conversations

☐ Difficulty remembering the date and/or year

☐ Temporarily forgetting the names of people close to them, such as friends and acquaintances

☐ Problems remembering where things are, such as misplacing keys or shoes; misplaced items may be found in strange places, such as kitchen items in the bedroom

☐ Getting lost more frequently, even on familiar routes such as the one from home to work

☐ Difficulty remembering traveling to a specific place or remembering why they are there

☐ Problems making decisions

☐ Demonstrating impaired reasoning and poor judgment

☐ Difficulty solving basic math problems

☐ Problems balancing a checkbook and difficulties in managing finances

☐ Difficulty recognizing financial scams

☐ Problems following directions, such as following a recipe or navigating to a new location

☐ Using several words or overly complex words to describe something simple

☐ Occasionally forgetting the correct word for something common, such as a clock

☐ Trouble expressing thoughts clearly and logically

☐ Frequently repeating stories or questions

☐ Recognizable personality changes

☐ Recognizable mood changes

☐ Problems with vision and depth perception

In the mild stage of Alzheimer's disease, symptoms often come and go, with the individual experiencing periods of forgetfulness intermingled with periods of lucidity. Sometimes, the mildness of these symptoms causes friends and family members to pass off the memory loss as a normal sign of aging. However, Alzheimer's disease is not a normal part of aging, and the pattern of memory loss can often help distinguish between normal aging and Alzheimer's disease.

Checklist: Differentiating between normal aging and Alzheimer's disease

☐ With normal aging, an individual may forget the name of an acquaintance they met recently or an individual they knew years ago; an individual with Alzheimer's disease will have trouble remembering the names and faces of their close family members and friends.

☐ With normal aging, an individual may get lost in an unfamiliar location; an individual with Alzheimer's disease will get lost traveling in familiar locations, such as between work and home or between home and the grocery store.

☐ With normal aging, an individual may repeat a question that they asked a few hours or days ago; an individual with Alzheimer's disease will repeatedly ask the same question within a few minutes.

☐ With normal aging, an individual might forget part of an experience or event that took place a year ago; an individual with Alzheimer's disease will forget that a recent event (e.g., within the last week) even took place.

☐ With normal aging, an individual who forgets something will likely remember it later; an individual with Alzheimer's disease will likely never realize that they forgot something at all.

☐ With normal aging, an individual might lose or misplace items but will be able to retrace their steps to find them; an individual with Alzheimer's disease will be unable to trace their steps to find lost or misplaced items.

☐ With normal aging, an individual will easily remember how to do something after a verbal or written reminder; an individual with Alzheimer's disease will have trouble following directions even if they used to do the task easily.

☐ With normal aging, making notes is a useful way to help the individual remember; individuals with Alzheimer's disease gradually benefit less from simple memory aids.

- [ ] With normal aging, an individual might miss a monthly payment once in a while; an individual with Alzheimer's disease will be unable to manage a budget and may forget that they have bills to pay.

- [ ] With normal aging, an individual might have trouble remembering a word; an individual with Alzheimer's disease will have trouble carrying on a conversation.

- [ ] With normal aging, an individual might make a bad decision once in a while; an individual with Alzheimer's disease will continually demonstrate poor judgment and decision making.

- [ ] With normal aging, an individual may take longer than normal to do an advanced task, such as program the DVR; an individual with Alzheimer's disease will forget how to do a simple task, such as brushing their teeth.

- [ ] With normal aging, an individual will be able to provide their own hygiene care, even if it is slower than normal; an individual with Alzheimer's disease will eventually be unable to provide their own hygiene care.

- [ ] With normal aging, the aging individual will be worried about their memory loss; an individual with Alzheimer's disease will likely not even realize that they are having memory problems.

If you recognize some of the symptoms of Alzheimer's disease in your loved one, or if your loved one has been diagnosed with Alzheimer's disease, the prognosis for your loved one at this early stage involves a steady worsening of symptoms, but the most difficult road is yet to come.

Checklist: Prognosis at stage 1

- [ ] Alzheimer's disease is generally diagnosed at this stage, and doctors may prescribe medications or lifestyle changes to slow the progression of the disease.

- [ ] Memory problems and other stage 1 symptoms will slowly become more noticeable.

- [ ] Individuals in stage 1 can generally still live alone, although they may need increasing help as they progress through the stage. Family and friends should help their loved one maintain independence for as long as possible. (See *Home Care, Long-Term Care, Memory Care Units, and Other Living Arrangements* for more information on maintaining functional independence for your loved one.)

☐ Safety concerns at stage 1 are minimal compared to other stages, but due to poor judgment and the possibility of getting lost, individuals in stage 1 should be monitored for worsening symptoms and dangerous behaviors. (See *Home Safety Checklist Guide and Caregiver Resources for Medication Safety, Driving, and Wandering* to learn more about maintaining your loved one's safety.)

☐ Depression is common after the initial diagnosis, and loved ones should watch for symptoms of depression, including feelings of hopelessness or helplessness, loss of interest in hobbies, fatigue, social withdrawal, changes in appetite, changes in sleep patterns, and thoughts of suicide. (Again, see *Home Safety Checklist Guide* for more information.)

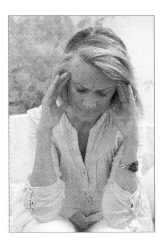

☐ An increase in anxiety may be present due to the worsening of symptoms.

Frequently, the most difficult part of stage 1 Alzheimer's disease is adjusting emotionally to the diagnosis and helping your loved one prepare for the future by getting their legal affairs in order. (See *Advance Directives, Durable Power of Attorney, Wills, and Other Legal Considerations* for more about legal issues.) For family and friends, watching your loved one slowly deteriorate can be emotionally draining, but you should take advantage of this stage by spending as much quality time with your loved one as you can before they begin to forget who you are and who they are.

Stage 2: Moderate

Stage 2 is the moderate stage of Alzheimer's disease. During this stage, symptoms become much more pronounced, with greater memory loss and mood changes taking place. The moderate stage of the disease is the longest and could continue for several years, with symptoms getting more severe as the individual ages. Individuals in this stage will likely need more help from caregivers, in-home assistants, and doctors (see *Home Care, Long-Term Care, Memory Care Units, and Other Living Arrangements*). Although called "moderate," this stage of Alzheimer's actually presents numerous and increasing difficulties to your loved one that will limit independent function.

Checklist: Symptoms of stage 2

☐ Progressive worsening of Stage 1 symptoms

☐ More apparent memory loss

☐ Difficulty recognizing loved ones and family

☐ Suspicion of strangers, even perceived strangers such as family and friends who your loved one no longer recognizes

☐ Problems remembering the day or year

☐ Repeating the same stories or experiences multiple times

☐ Making up past events because they cannot remember what actually happened

☐ Frequent periods of confusion

☐ More frequent wandering (see *Home Safety Checklist Guide and Caregiver Resources for Medication Safety, Driving, and Wandering*), which comes as a result of feeling disoriented or confused in once-familiar surroundings

☐ Increased restlessness, particularly late in the day (sometimes referred to as "sundowning")

☐ Difficulties with coordination while walking

☐ Difficulty dressing without assistance

☐ Wearing clothes that are not appropriate for the weather or occasion

☐ Displaying uncharacteristic behaviors such as refusing to change clothes or refusing to bathe; affected individuals may become belligerent or aggressive when forced to perform common hygiene tasks

☐ Difficulty performing tasks that have more than one step

- ☐ Difficulty with math and logic problems

- ☐ Increased difficulty reading or writing

- ☐ Difficulty bathing

- ☐ Eating problems

- ☐ Periods of incontinence

- ☐ Changes in sleeping habits, such as sleeping during the day and being awake at night

- ☐ Increased changes in personality, including aggression, paranoia, and depression

- ☐ Displaying inappropriate sexual behavior

- ☐ Increased agitation when encountering new situations

- ☐ Hoarding items, such as paper and shoelaces

- ☐ Visual hallucinations

- ☐ Auditory hallucinations

During stage 2, your loved one will need greater care and assistance on a daily basis, and they will gradually lose the capacity to live and travel independently. The following checklist details the prognosis for your loved one at stage 2 of Alzheimer's disease. (See *Home Safety Checklist Guide and Caregiver Resources for Medication Safety, Driving, and Wandering* for more on safety concerns such as wandering and driving safety. See *Home Care, Long-Term Care, Memory Care Units, and Other Living Arrangements* for more on home healthcare assistants, moving in with a caregiver, and long-term care.)

Checklist: Prognosis at stage 2

- ☐ Safety concerns for your loved one will increase.

- ☐ Due to wandering and confusion, your loved one will require increased observation.

☐ You loved one will need greater assistance with activities in and around the home, including activities of daily living (e.g., bathing, dressing, eating, etc.).

☐ Your loved one will become less able to do their own cooking and cleaning.

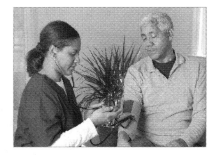

☐ Your loved one will lose the ability to drive based on safety reasons.

☐ Your loved one will likely require the help of home healthcare assistants.

☐ Periods of depression and anxiety may become more prevalent.

☐ If living alone, your loved one might need someone to move in with them; alternatively, your loved one might need to move in with a caregiver.

☐ Long-term care (e.g., assisted living or a memory care unit) might be considered if no in-home caregiver is available.

☐ In this stage, your loved one will have good days and bad days; near the end of stage 2, the bad days may be more prevalent.

☐ Toward the end of this stage, the progression of the disease may become more rapid.

☐ If medications have not yet been prescribed, your loved one's physician may prescribe medications to slow the progression of some symptoms before they become severe.

☐ Medications might be prescribed to treat behavioral symptoms. Some people experience debilitating side effects from the medications, which if present would necessitate stopping treatment.

Stage 2 of Alzheimer's disease is typically the longest and most difficult for caregivers, because caregivers often carry the entire burden of caring for their loved one on their own. In addition, the confusion brought on by memory loss may make your loved one difficult to handle in some situations. By the end of stage 2, many caregivers are unable to take care of their loved one on their own and will place their loved one in a long-term care facility such as a nursing home or memory care unit.

Stage 3: Severe

In the final stage of Alzheimer's disease, the severe stage, symptoms become very advanced. Individuals who progress to the final years of Alzheimer's disease generally lose the ability to move and communicate, making it necessary to have full-time care. The third stage can last anywhere from a few months to a year or more. The following checklist details the symptoms of severe Alzheimer's disease.

Checklist: Symptoms at stage 3

☐ Inability to recognize family, loved ones, places, or objects

☐ Loss of communication skills

☐ Increased time spent sleeping

☐ Marked decrease in thirst and appetite

☐ Inability to eat without assistance

☐ Difficulty swallowing

☐ Weight loss

☐ Increased aspiration (inhaling) of food and liquids into the lungs

☐ Increased risk of pneumonia, especially aspiration pneumonia

☐ Difficulty or inability to perform tasks related to self-care, such as dressing, bathing, toileting, etc.

☐ Loss of bladder and bowel control

☐ Increased frequency of urinary tract infections

☐ Decline in muscle strength and flexibility

☐ Difficulty walking unassisted

☐ Loss of muscle control in the neck, making it difficult to hold one's head up without help

☐ Loss of the ability to smile

☐ Elevated potential for seizures

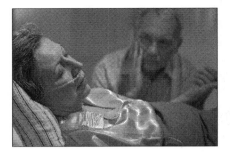

The prognosis of late-stage Alzheimer's disease is ultimately end-of-life care. In the early months of this stage, as symptoms begin to intensify, the goal will primarily be symptom management. However, as your loved one's condition worsens, the care will likely become preventative and palliative in nature. Palliative care includes making sure your loved one is comfortable (i.e., pain management) and has all of their basic needs provided (e.g., nutrition, water, hygiene care). Preventative care will generally focus on the prevention of complications, including urinary tract infections and pneumonia.

Checklist: Complications associated with end-stage Alzheimer's disease

Urinary tract infections (UTIs):

☐ UTIs result from dehydration, incomplete bladder emptying, and poor hygiene. They also result from catheter use, but catheter use is not recommended for controlling incontinence in individuals with Alzheimer's disease.

☐ UTIs are more common in women than in men, but both genders are at an increased risk as they age.

☐ UTIs in individuals with Alzheimer's disease do not present with the normal signs of infection, such as pain and fever.

☐ Typical signs of UTIs in individuals with Alzheimer's disease include increased confusion, agitation, withdrawal, decreased appetite, increased time spent sleeping, decreased balance control, increased incidence of falls, sudden decrease in the ability to perform tasks, and violent or odd behavior.

☐ UTIs can be diagnosed with a simple urine test.

☐ Antibiotics may be used to treat a UTI; if left untreated, the infection could cause serious medical complications.

☐ The presence of an infection such as a UTI can speed the progression of Alzheimer's disease.

Pneumonia:

☐ Pneumonia is a condition involving swelling or infection of the lungs or large airways that affects breathing.

☐ One of the most common types of pneumonia experienced by individuals with Alzheimer's disease is aspiration pneumonia.

☐ Aspiration pneumonia is common in individuals who experience difficulty swallowing, causing them to inhale substances such as food, saliva, liquids, or vomit into their lungs; this process is called aspiration.

☐ Aspiration pneumonia can lead to death for individuals with Alzheimer's disease. Even so, many doctors hesitate to suggest antibiotics for these patients because they are usually administered in a hospital setting with the use of an IV, and they may cause your loved one increased discomfort. In addition, individuals with Alzheimer's disease tend to pull out IVs, and they often require sedation due to extreme agitation.

☐ Another common cause of pneumonia in individuals with Alzheimer's disease is influenza, or the flu. Therefore, the CDC recommends that individuals with Alzheimer's disease, as well as their caregivers, receive the flu vaccine each year.

☐ Along with the flu vaccine, individuals with Alzheimer's disease may want to get a pneumonia vaccine, although this does not prevent pneumonia related to aspiration.

The final stage of Alzheimer's disease will end in death for your loved one. Although loved ones often feel the need to avoid this issue, it is the inevitable consequence of Alzheimer's disease. As your loved one progresses through the three stages of Alzheimer's disease, find comfort in spending time with them, even it if is difficult to see your loved one gradually slip away from being the person you once knew. Treasure every moment you have together. I remember taking my dad out to dinner during the early stages of his disease, and I would get really frustrated with him. He would drink his salad dressing, eat his soup with his fingers, and not be able to have a coherent conversation. Then it occurred to me that every day would be better than the next one, so I had to treasure these moments even if my dad had only a lucid sentence or two. Once he got to the point that he could no longer speak, I was grateful that I had changed my attitude and enjoyed those earlier times with him.

Early-Onset Alzheimer's Disease

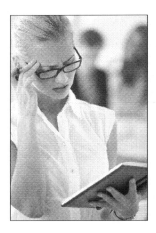

Although Alzheimer's disease most frequently affects individuals who are over age 60, a subset of individuals will develop early-onset Alzheimer's disease, which is differentiated from classic Alzheimer's disease by the age at which it manifests. For individuals with early-onset Alzheimer's disease, symptoms typically begin when they are in their 40s or 50s. In rare cases, symptoms will appear when individuals are in their late 20s or 30s. Early-onset Alzheimer's disease is often genetic, passed down to children from their parents and grandparents, but it can also be sporadic and unexplained. Approximately 200,000 individuals in the United States have early-onset Alzheimer's disease, but many go undiagnosed or misdiagnosed for a long time. Due to the perception that Alzheimer's disease only affects individuals in their mid- to late 60s or older, many people who have memory loss symptoms in their 30s and 40s are diagnosed with stress disorders or other ailments. Thus, these individuals do not get the proper care and treatment they require.

Early-onset Alzheimer's disease has essentially the same symptoms and characteristics as classic Alzheimer's disease. However, many people perceive that individuals with early-onset Alzheimer's disease progress through the disease more quickly than those who develop the disease later in life. This perception has not been confirmed through rigorous scientific studies, and it may stem from the fact that individuals with early-onset Alzheimer's disease often enter long-term care facilities much earlier in the course of the disease simply because their spouse and family are younger and are unable to provide daily, full-time care due to the responsibilities of work and raising children.

Early-onset Alzheimer's disease can be especially hard on families and spouses because it is often unexpected and occurs in the individual's prime years. Your loved one may still have children living at home, is likely to still be working full time, and could even be in the early years of a marriage. In addition, individuals who develop early-onset Alzheimer's disease may have a harder time finding a full-time caregiver because their spouse has to work full-time and their children are not grown and are thus unable to handle the responsibility.

For example, when we moved my father to a nursing home, we met a fellow resident named Jan (name has been changed to protect her privacy). Jan was 35 years old and had been diagnosed three years prior. She had three young children that she sometimes knew and sometimes did not know. Her husband could not take the emotional or financial stress and moved away from the situation. Jan's mom ended up taking care of the kids and visiting Jan on a daily basis. Jan's mom told me that it was difficult to find a nursing home that would take Jan because of her age. Nursing homes were concerned about liability and sexual abuse of Jan. Finally, my father's nursing home signed off on accepting Jan. The complications associated with providing care for younger individuals often make coping with early-onset Alzheimer's disease more difficult than coping with classic Alzheimer's disease that develops later in life. The following checklist provides some tips for coping with early-onset Alzheimer's disease.

Checklist: Coping with early-onset Alzheimer's disease

- ☐ Encourage your loved one to ask for help, especially from their spouse and/or family.

- ☐ Recommend that your loved one consult a counselor or therapist to communicate openly about their fears regarding the disease.

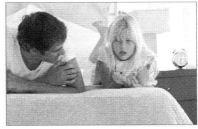

- ☐ Recommend that your loved one and family join a community support group for individuals and families dealing with Alzheimer's disease.

- ☐ Look into couples counseling if your loved one is worried about changes in their marriage relationship.

- ☐ Encourage your loved one and their spouse to find activities they can still enjoy together.

☐ Recommend that your loved one discuss the disease and the changes that may take place with their children. Explain what is happening in terms the child will understand.

☐ Encourage the child or children to talk about their feelings and fears openly.

☐ Involve young children in therapy or counseling sessions so that they better understand what is happening to their parent.

☐ Encourage your loved one to spend as much time with their children as possible.

☐ Suggest that your loved one write notes or cards or make a video to give to each child on special occasions in the future, such as birthdays, graduations, and weddings. This should be done early in the disease when your loved one still has the mental capacity to do so.

☐ Encourage your loved one to talk with his or her employer to arrange different shifts and/or a different position, if necessary.

☐ Recommend that your loved one decrease their hours at work if they are feeling overwhelmed.

☐ Research the Americans with Disabilities Act (ADA) to see whether your loved one is entitled to any benefits.

If you are a friend or close family member (who is not a spouse or child) of someone with early-onset Alzheimer's disease, providing support and caregiving relief will be a huge blessing to the family. Watching children for a few hours, doing grocery shopping or other errands for the family, providing a meal, listening to fears and frustrations, or spending time with your loved one with Alzheimer's disease are all ways that you can help lift the burden of this disease.

Treatment

Currently, no drug therapies are available that can cure Alzheimer's disease; therefore, the major goal of treatment is slowing the progression of Alzheimer's disease's and extending the individual's quality of life. Primarily, efforts at slowing the progress of Alzheimer's disease involve using FDA-approved medications to slow your loved one's mental decline and treat the specific symptoms afflicting your loved one. In addition to drug therapies, your loved one might want to try various natural and alternative therapies; however, you should explore these alternatives with caution, because dietary supplements and medical foods are not subject to FDA approval and regulation.

Many non-drug options exist for managing the behavioral symptoms of Alzheimer's disease. These symptoms include difficulties in performing normal daily activities (e.g., cooking, paying bills, shopping, etc.), behavioral issues (e.g., anger, depression, aggression, or problems with self-expression), and problems with self-care (e.g., bathing, dressing, grooming, etc.). Options for addressing these symptoms include communication strategies that caregivers can use to help loved ones with Alzheimer's disease better cope with the disease, therapeutic regimens that assist loved ones with daily functioning, and routines of diet and exercise that may help your loved one slow their physical and mental decline. However, do not neglect drug therapies, which may be necessary if other approaches fail to effectively manage your loved one's behavioral problems.

Prescription Medications

Medications for Alzheimer's disease can generally be classified into two broad groups: medications that combat the activity of the disease itself (the process of cognitive decline) and medications that combat the behavioral symptoms that arise during the course of the disease (depression, anxiety, and other mood and behavioral problems). The FDA has approved drugs in two different classes to treat cognitive symptoms associated with Alzheimer's disease: cholinesterase inhibitors and NMDA antagonists.

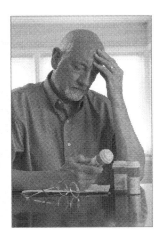

Checklist: Facts about cholinesterase inhibitors

General facts:

☐ Cholinesterase (pronounced koh-lin-'ess-ter-ace) inhibitors work by preserving high levels of acetylcholine (pronounced uh-see-til-'koh-leen or 'a-seh-teel-'koh-leen) in the brain. As neurons become damaged and die, the levels of acetylcholine in the brain decrease. Cholinesterase inhibitors prevent the breakdown of acetylcholine, thus prolonging their actions and enhancing neuron signaling in the brain.

☐ The three cholinesterase inhibitors on the market are donepezil (Aricept), rivastigmine (Exelon), and galantamine (Razadyne).

☐ A fourth cholinesterase inhibitor, tacrine (Cognex), is available but is rarely prescribed because of severe side effects.

☐ Cholinesterase inhibitors are usually prescribed in the mild and moderate stages of Alzheimer's disease.

☐ Aricept is the only cholinesterase inhibitor approved for use in severe Alzheimer's disease.

☐ Cholinesterase inhibitors only work for about 50% of the individuals that take them, and they work to varying degrees in these individuals.

☐ For those individuals who see positive effects from cholinesterase inhibitors, the effects only last for six months to one year before the disease begins to progress again.

☐ Cholinesterase inhibitors only delay the decline of mental function for individuals with Alzheimer's disease. They do not halt the effects of Alzheimer's disease.

Therapeutic effects:

Cholinesterase inhibitors improve, stabilize, or cause a less than expected decline in each of the following:

☐ Cognition

☐ Memory problems

☐ Ability to perform activities of daily living

☐ Ability to form correct judgments

☐ Ability to think and communicate clearly

☐ Severity of dementia

- [ ] Behavioral problems

- [ ] Global functioning

- [ ] Deposition of amyloid in the brain (Aricept only)

Side effects:

- [ ] Nausea and vomiting

- [ ] Diarrhea

- [ ] Weight loss

- [ ] Loss of appetite

- [ ] Sleep disturbances

With regard to side effects, note that Aricept is generally tolerated better than Exelon and Razadyne.

Checklist: Facts about NMDA antagonists

General facts:

- [ ] N-methyl D-aspartate (NMDA) antagonists regulate the activity of glutamate in the brain; glutamate is involved in learning and memory. Damaged neurons release excess glutamate, speeding up the destruction of nearby neurons. NMDA antagonists partially block the effects of glutamate, thus protecting neurons.

- [ ] The only NMDA antagonist approved for use in Alzheimer's disease is memantine (Namenda).

- [ ] Namenda can be prescribed in both the moderate and severe stages of Alzheimer's disease.

- [ ] Because they have different mechanisms of action, Namenda can be prescribed along with a cholinesterase inhibitor to produce greater results.

- [ ] The benefits of Namenda are similar to those of cholinesterase inhibitors in that the effects are temporary, only delaying the progression of Alzheimer's disease.

Therapeutic effects:

☐ Improves memory, attention span, and reasoning skills

☐ Improves language capabilities

☐ Improves the ability to perform simple tasks

Side effects:

☐ Confusion

☐ Dizziness

☐ Headaches

☐ Constipation

In addition to drugs approved specifically to treat Alzheimer's disease, many physicians will prescribe medications to decrease behavioral symptoms associated with Alzheimer's disease. However, these drugs are usually only prescribed if non-drug behavioral modification therapies are ineffective. A brief list of behavioral drugs is included in the following checklist, including the types of behavioral problems that they treat.

Checklist: Drugs used to treat behavioral problems

☐ **Depression and anxiety.** Antidepressants include citalopram (Celexa), mirtazapine (Remeron), sertraline (Zoloft), and others.

☐ **Aggression.** Anticonvulsants include sodium valproate (Depakote), carbamazepine (Tegretol), oxcarbazepine (Trileptal), and others.

☐ **Sleep aids.** Sleep aids include zolpidem (Ambien), eszopiclone (Lunesta), zaleplon (Sonata), and others. These drugs may increase confusion and increase the likelihood of falls.

☐ **Agitation.** Anti-anxiety drugs include lorazepam (Ativan), clonazepam (Klonopin), and others. These drugs may cause sleepiness, dizziness, falls, and confusion.

☐ **Paranoia and hallucinations.** Antipsychotics include risperidone (Risperdal), quetiapine (Seroquel), olanzapine (Zyprexa), and others. These drugs may have serious side effects, including risk of death in older individuals with dementia.

☐ **Drugs that should NOT be given to individuals with Alzheimer's disease.** Because of the risk of serious side effects, including increased confusion, ipratropium (Atrovent), ipratropium and albuterol (Combivent), ipratropium and albuterol (DuoNeb), and tiotropium (Spiriva) should not be given to individuals with Alzheimer's disease.

Because the side effects of some of these drugs may be severe, physicians typically prescribe them in dosages just high enough to ease symptoms, carefully adjusting the dosage to fit the patient's current needs. The following checklist highlights some important things to keep in mind concerning drug treatment for your loved one.

Checklist: Considerations for drug treatment

☐ Ensure that your loved one's physician and pharmacist know all of the medications your loved one is currently taking, including alternative medicines and over-the-counter drugs. Because the interactions of different medications taken together can produce side effects, the doctor and pharmacist both need to have a complete and accurate list of your loved one's medications.

☐ As your loved one's condition declines, they might need to be reminded to take their medications at the proper times and dosage levels, and you may need to give them their medications yourself and watch them take the medications to ensure that they aren't skipping doses.

☐ Buy a pillbox (available at the drugstore) to organize the pills for each day into separate compartments in the box. This keeps all your loved one's pills in one place while also making it easier for your loved one to manage when and how much of each pill to take.

☐ Find out everything you can from your loved one's physician and pharmacist regarding each type of medication your loved one is taking, and record the answers where you will have them ready for easy reference.

☐ Questions to ask concerning each of your loved one's medications include why the drug was prescribed, what the positive effects should be, what the daily dosage is, when the drug should be taken, what the side effects are, how the drug should be administered (such as if it needs to be taken with food), and what effects its interaction with other drugs might produce.

You or your loved might also ask your loved one's physician about the use of Vitamin E (in its alpha-tocopherol form). In a 2014 study, individuals with mild or moderate Alzheimer's disease who took high doses of Vitamin E had a slowed functional decline. Vitamin E is an antioxidant; antioxidants may produce brain health benefits by protecting brain cells from damage. However, high doses of Vitamin E can also be harmful, increasing the risk of death for some people who take medications to lower their cholesterol. For this reason, your loved one should never take Vitamin E to manage the symptoms of Alzheimer's disease without a prescription from their physician.

Alternative Treatments

In addition to prescription medications, alternative treatments—such as herbal remedies, foods thought to produce specific health benefits (also known as "medical foods"), and dietary supplements—are also available for your loved to try. However, be sure to ask your loved one's physician about all such remedies before trying them. The FDA demands that a high standard of scientific research be met when it examines prescription drugs for approval, but alternative treatments do not need to meet this standard because they are not subject to FDA approval.

Sellers of alternative remedies often base claims for their efficacy and safety on testimonials and endorsements. These are usually claims from a few individuals that aren't necessarily typical of the general population or even factual, and the companies that provide these remedies may not have information about or disclose potential side effects. In the case of dietary supplements, their purity might be questionable (the FDA does not regulate how these supplements are produced), and they might have adverse interactions with drugs your loved one's physician has prescribed. In the case of medical foods, some were intended as prescription drugs but ran into problems during the clinical trials, so their developers chose to market them as foods or supplements to avoid obstacles that would prevent FDA approval.

For these reasons, you and your loved one should approach all such alternatives with caution.

The following checklist summarizes the alternative treatments available that are thought by some to have potential health benefits for people with Alzheimer's disease. This list also summarizes what evidence exists for their effectiveness, if any. Again, approach these with caution and use only with the advice and endorsement of your loved one's physician. It might be tempting when faced with Alzheimer's disease to try anything that could possibly be of benefit, but for the sake of your loved one, be judicious with respect to alternative treatments.

Checklist: Effectiveness of alternative treatments for Alzheimer's disease

Herbal remedies:

☐ **Ginkgo biloba.** The plant extract ginkgo biloba has been used in traditional Chinese medical practice for its antioxidant and anti-inflammatory properties, and in Europe today this extract is being used to ease symptoms related to various neurological conditions. Several studies have investigated the benefits of ginkgo biloba for individuals with Alzheimer's disease. Some of the trials proved inconclusive, some showed no effect, some showed a small effect that is likely clinically insignificant, and some showed a modest effect. Overall, the evidence is weak that ginkgo biloba provides some cognitive benefits for individuals with Alzheimer's disease.

Medical foods:

☐ **Caprylic acid.** Caprylic acid, which can be found in coconut oil and is marketed under the name Axona as a medical food, is a fat that the body breaks down into ketone bodies. The belief that caprylic acid can help people with Alzheimer's disease derives from the idea that ketone bodies work as an alternative fuel source for brain cells that can no longer convert glucose, their main source of energy, into the energy they need to function. Although caprylic acid was tested in Phase II clinical trials under the name Ketasyn with promising results, it did not undergo Phase III trials, and no large studies have indicated Axona's effectiveness in treating Alzheimer's disease. Subsequently, the company that produces Axona has been issued a warning by the FDA that Axona does not meet the criteria for a medical food because evidence substantiating their claims that it can treat Alzheimer's disease is insufficient. Some individuals use coconut oil as a cheaper source of caprylic acid, but no clinical testing has ever been done to investigate the effectiveness of coconut oil in Alzheimer's disease.

☐ **Tramiprosate.** Tramiprosate is a medical food that is a modified form of taurine, an amino acid that occurs naturally in seaweed. Although a large Phase III clinical study tested the potential use of tramiprosate as a treatment for Alzheimer's disease, because the data was inconclusive, the manufacturer elected to market tramiprosate as a medical food instead of getting it approved as a prescription drug by the FDA. Consequently, the manufacturer has not proven the effectiveness of tramiprosate.

Dietary supplements:

☐ **Acetyl-L-carnitine.** Acetyl-L-carnitine (ALC) regulates energy and lipid metabolism, has neuroprotective effects, and can be converted to acetylcholine. Two large studies indicated that no overall benefit is seen in Alzheimer's disease. However, it appeared to have a small benefit for younger patients and may be beneficial for individuals with early-onset Alzheimer's disease. Several small studies have confirmed that ALC does not appear to benefit individuals with Alzheimer's disease beyond the mild stage.

☐ **Coenzyme Q10.** The antioxidant Coenzyme Q10, also called ubiquinone, is a compound that the body produces naturally and that plays a role in normal cell reactions. No studies for its effectiveness in treating Alzheimer's disease have been conducted, although tests of the synthetic version, idebenone, have shown that it has no benefit for people with Alzheimer's disease. Additionally, Coenzyme Q10 could be harmful if taken in high doses, and information about dosage requirements is severely limited.

☐ **"Coral" calcium.** Coral calcium comes from the shells of the organisms that form coral reefs. Despite bold marketing claims that this type of calcium carbonate can cure Alzheimer's disease, coral calcium does not cure Alzheimer's disease. Both the FDA and the Federal Trade Commission (FTC) have filed formal complaints against the marketers and distributors of coral calcium because their claims are entirely unsupported by any credible scientific evidence, and making such claims without scientific evidence is illegal. An individual may take calcium supplements to promote bone health, but instead of coral calcium, calcium supplements should be prepared in a purified form by a reputable manufacturer.

☐ **Huperzine A.** A moss extract called huperzine A, another supplement that is used in traditional Chinese medicine, possesses similar properties to cholinesterase inhibitors, the prescription drugs used to treat Alzheimer's disease. Accordingly, huperzine A has been promoted as a viable alternative means of treating Alzheimer's disease. However, a large clinical study conducted by the Alzheimer's Disease Cooperative Study (ADCS) showed no benefit to taking huperzine A as a treatment for Alzheimer's disease.

☐ **Omega 3 fatty acids.** Omega-3s such as docosahexaneoic acid (DHA) and eicosapentaenoic acid (EPA) are polyunsaturated fats. Although some research has found a possible connection between taking high amounts of omega-3s and reducing the risk of dementia and cognitive decline, the results of two major studies concerning the effectiveness of omega-3s in this regard are inconclusive. The scientific opinion is that the evidence for omega-3s as an effective treatment for Alzheimer's disease is not sufficient. FDA recommendations regarding intake of DHA or EPA are no more than 3 grams a day, no more than 2 of which can come from supplements.

☐ **Phosphatidylserine.** A kind of lipid called phosphatidylserine is the primary component of the membranes surrounding nerve cells, and because Alzheimer's disease causes degeneration of nerve cells, phosphatidylserine has been considered as a treatment for Alzheimer's disease. Although early trials delivered results that seemed promising, they also involved the brain cells of cows, and concerns about mad cow disease put a stop to these trials in the 90s. Since then, supplements that contain phosphatidylserine have been derived from soy extracts. Although the FDA allows these supplements to include a qualified claim regarding their effectiveness, the FDA's conclusion is that the evidence for this claim is scant, and the scientific opinion recommends against use of phosphatidylserine.

☐ **Piracetam.** Piracetam is a derivative of gamma-aminobutyric acid, a chemical that inhibits neuron transmissions. Several small studies with piracetam have shown no overall benefit in individuals with Alzheimer's disease or other forms of dementia. However, individual studies indicated improvement, although the definition of improvement was not given. Overall, studies indicate that piracetam is not beneficial for treating Alzheimer's disease.

Regardless of the treatment options that you or your loved one would like to pursue, all treatments should be discussed with your loved one's physician and only taken under the care and guidance of a doctor. Drug and supplement interactions and side effects may cause your loved one to stop taking some medications, but stopping some medications suddenly can lead to withdrawal symptoms. Therefore, discuss any concerns with a physician before starting or stopping any medications or supplements.

Clinical Trials

The National Institute on Aging (NIA), one of the National Institutes of Health, is the federal agency tasked with taking the lead on Alzheimer's disease research. The NIA supports efforts (involving everything from early Phase I trials through Phase III trials that test actual effectiveness) to study drugs and other types of interventions (such as exercise) to see whether they may slow the progress of Alzheimer's disease, ease its symptoms, or prevent it entirely. Prevention trials are a strong current focus of the NIA's efforts.

Many clinical trials are currently being conducted to examine and test the efficacy of various potential pharmacological treatments for Alzheimer's disease and other forms of dementia. All new medications must pass exhaustive laboratory tests involving first animals and then humans before they may be approved and sold as prescription drugs. The clinical trials are just the first step. When they have concluded, a drug company applies to the FDA, which in cooperation with an independent medical panel conducts stringent examinations to determine whether the drug is safe and effective enough to merit approval as a prescription drug.

Clinical trials are conducted all across the country. If there is a clinical trial in your area, should your loved one participate? The following checklist examines the potential problems and benefits involved with this. Remember that although participating in a clinical trial may or may not directly benefit your loved one, such trials are essential to ultimately finding effective treatments for Alzheimer's disease. No cure for Alzheimer's disease can be found without them.

Checklist: Participation in a clinical trial

☐ Most often, clinical trials test treatments for the early stage of Alzheimer's disease.

☐ The subject may only be given a *placebo*, which is a pill or treatment that looks like the real treatment but contains no active drugs. This is a routine part of clinical testing; the effects of the real drug are measured against the placebo. If there is no real difference from the placebo, then the drug is probably not effective.

☐ Clinical trials take a long time to complete.

☐ A clinical trial can be time-consuming for caregivers. Even if the trial doesn't involve travel, it could involve multiple appointments each week, the need for ongoing monitoring of changes, etc.

☐ Most clinical trials show minimal differences between the control group (the group taking the placebo) and the treatment group (the group taking the actual drug). In other words, most clinical trials show that the treatment being tested is ineffective.

Because clinical trials are time-consuming and intensive, your loved one should carefully consider making this commitment and what that might mean for how they want to spend the time they have left with their families, how advanced Alzheimer's disease is for them, and if they are willing to take the risks associated with unproven medications.

Conclusion

Alzheimer's disease is different for every person who has it based on individual factors of genetics, lifestyle, and environment. Alzheimer's disease affects different people in different ways, and it progresses at different rates. However, Alzheimer's disease is commonly divided into three main stages—mild, moderate, and severe— and although not everyone with the disease experiences the symptoms of each stage in exactly the same order or the same way, people with the disease generally progress from a mild stage where the disease is first diagnosed, through a moderate stage where individuals slowly lose their ability to function independently, and finally to a severe stage where individuals must receive full-time care. The severe stage ends in death. Although no known treatments can cure or halt Alzheimer's disease, the disease's progress may be slowed and its symptoms, both of cognitive decline and increasing behavioral problems, may be eased through the use of prescription medications and therapies. With the help of your loved one's physician, explore diet, exercise, drug therapies, and non-drug therapies as ways to maintain quality of life and independent function for your loved one as long as possible.

ABOUT THE AUTHORS

Laura Town

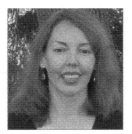

Laura Town has authored numerous publications of special interest to the aging population. She has expertise in the field of finance as a co-author on *Finance: Foundations of Financial Institutions and Management* published by John Wiley and Sons, and she has contributed to several online nursing courses and texts. She has also written for the American Medical Writers Association, and her work has been published by the American Society of Journalists and Authors. As an editor, Laura has worked with Pearson Education, Prentice Hall, McGraw-Hill Higher Education, John Wiley and Sons, and the University of Pennsylvania to create both on-ground and online courses and texts. She is currently the President of the Indiana chapter of the American Medical Writers Association.

Karen Kassel

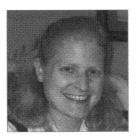

Karen Kassel received her Ph.D. in pharmacology from the Department of Pharmacology and Experimental Neurosciences at the University of Nebraska Medical Center in Omaha, where she was the recipient of an American Heart Association fellowship and several regional and national awards for her research on G protein-coupled receptor signaling in airways. She then pursued post-doctoral research projects at the University of North Carolina–Chapel Hill and the University of Kansas Medical Center, again receiving fellowships from the PhRMA Foundation and the American Heart Association, respectively. She has published research in the *American Journal of Pathology*, *Journal of Biological Chemistry*, and *Journal of Pharmacology and Experimental Therapeutics*. In 2012, Karen joined the editorial staff at WilliamsTown Communications, an editing firm that specializes in educational products for undergraduate- and graduate-level students. At WTC, Karen specializes in producing educational products related to the sciences and healthcare. In addition, Karen recently became board-certified for editing life sciences (BELS-certified).

A NOTE FROM THE AUTHORS

Thank you for purchasing our book! Worldwide, over 40 million people suffer from Alzheimer's disease, and that number is expected to increase significantly within the next 15 years. In the United States, over five million people have the disease, and that is expected to triple by the year 2050.

Despite these large numbers, you may feel alone. I (Laura) know that when I started caring for my father, who had early-onset Alzheimer's disease, I felt alone. Although my father has passed away, I am haunted by what he suffered and how difficult it was to care for him. However, now I know that there are people, resources, and organizations that can help others going through this same struggle.

We recognize that caregivers have emotional, physical, and financial challenges. We hope that the information in the *Alzheimer's Roadmap* series will ease some of your stress. The symptoms and treatments discussed in this book will help you prepare for the road ahead and understand options that are available to you and your loved one. In addition, we have included resources at the end of each book to provide additional information to help you through this process.

If you have any questions for us, feel free to post them on Laura Town's Amazon Author Central page or reach out to either author via twitter: @laurawtown and @KarenKassel1. We would appreciate it if you would take the time to review our book on Amazon, as our book's visibility on Amazon depends on reviews.

More Titles from Laura Town and Karen Kassel

☐ *Long-Term Care Insurance, Power of Attorney, Wealth Management, and Other First Steps*

☐ *Advance Directives, Durable Power of Attorney, Wills, and Other Legal Considerations*

☐ *Paying for Healthcare and Other Financial Considerations*

☐ *Home Safety Checklist Guide and Caregiver Resources for Medication Safety, Driving, and Wandering*

☐ *Home Care, Long-Term Care, Memory Care Units, and Other Living Arrangements*

☐ *Caregiver Resources for Helping with Activities of Daily Living*

☐ *Nutrition for Brain Health: Fighting Dementia*

☐ *Caregiver Resources: From Independence to a Memory Care Unit*

(This book combines information from *Home Safety Checklist Guide and Caregiver Resources for Medication Safety, Driving, and Wandering* and information from *Home Care, Long-Term Care, Memory Care Units, and Other Living Arrangements.*)

RESOURCES

Information about Alzheimer's Disease

Alzheimer's Association
225 N. Michigan Avenue, Floor 17
Chicago, IL 60601-7633
Phone: 800-272-3900
Fax: 866-699-1246
Email: info@alz.org
Website: http://www.alz.org

Alzheimer's Disease Education and Referral (ADEAR) Center
P.O. Box 8250
Silver Spring, MD 20907-8250
Phone: 800-438-4380
Website: http://www.nia.nih.gov/alzheimers
*Includes information related to current clinical trials

Alzheimer's Foundation of America
322 Eighth Avenue, 7th Floor
New York, NY 10001
Phone: 866-232-8484
Fax: 646-638-1546
Website: http://www.alzfdn.org

Fisher Center for Alzheimer's Research Foundation
110 East 42nd Street, 16th Floor
New York, NY 10017
Phone: 800-ALZINFO (259-4636)
Fax: 212-915-1319
Email: info@alzinfo.org
Website: http://www.alzinfo.org/
*Includes resource locator for physicians and treatment centers for Alzheimer's disease

U.S. Department of Health and Human Services
Alzheimer's disease webpage: http://www.alzheimers.gov/index.html

Information about the Americans with Disabilities Act

United States Department of Labor
200 Constitution Avenue NW
Washington, DC 20210
Phone: 866-4-USA-DOL (487-2365)
Email: webmaster@dol.gov
Website: http://www.dol.gov/dol/topic/disability/ada.htm

U.S. Equal Employment Opportunity Commission
Phone: 800-669-4000
Website: http://www.eeoc.gov/eeoc/publications/fs-ada.cfm

Other

Other books in the Alzheimer's Roadmap series

- *Long-Term Care Insurance, Power of Attorney, Wealth Management, and Other First Steps*

- *Advance Directives, Durable Power of Attorney, Wills, and Other Legal Considerations*

- *Paying for Healthcare and Other Financial Considerations*

- *Home Safety Checklist Guide and Caregiver Resources for Medication Safety, Driving, and Wandering*

- *Home Care, Long-Term Care, Memory Care Units, and Other Living Arrangements*

- *Caregiver Resources for Helping with Activities of Daily Living*

- *Nutrition for Brain Health: Fighting Dementia*

- *Caregiver Resources: From Independence to a Memory Care Unit*

  (This book combines information from *Home Safety Checklist Guide and Caregiver Resources for Medication Safety, Driving, and Wandering* and information from *Home Care, Long-Term Care, Memory Care Units, and Other Living Arrangements*.)

REFERENCE LIST

Alzheimer's Association. (2015). Retrieved from http://www.alz.org/

Alzheimer's Disease International. (2015). Retrieved from http://www.alz.co.uk/

Alzheimer's Foundation of America. (2015). Retrieved from http://www.alzfdn.org/index.htm

Alzheimer's Society. (2015). Retrieved from http://www.alzheimers.org.uk/site/index.php

Alzheimer's Society Canada. (2015). Retrieved from http://www.alzheimer.ca/en

American Board of Professional Psychology. (n.d.). Clinical neuropsychology. Retrieved from http://www.abpp.org/i4a/pages/index.cfm?pageid=3304

American Neuropsychiatric Society. (n.d.). Neuropsychiatry has two referents: A scientific field and a medical subspecialty. Retrieved from http://www.anpaonline.org/what-is-neuropsychiatry-behavioral-neurology

Colovic, M.B., Krstic, D.Z., Lazarevic-Pasti, T.D., Bondzic, A.M., & Vasic, V.M. (2013). Acetylcholinesterase inhibitors: Pharmacology and toxicology. *Current Neuropharmacology, 11*(3), 315–335.

Fisher Center for Alzheimer's Research Foundation. (2014). Retrieved from http://www.alzinfo.org/

Hill, C. (2014). What's the difference between Alzheimer's and normal age-related memory loss? Retrieved from http://alzheimers.about.com/od/whatisalzheimer1/f/NormalAging.htm

Johns Hopkins Medicine. (n.d.) Early-onset Alzheimer's disease. Retrieved from http://www.hopkinsmedicine.org/healthlibrary/conditions/nervous_system_disorders/early-onset_alzheimers_disease_134,63/

Kelley, B.J., & Knopman, D.S. (2008). Alternative medicine and Alzheimer's disease. *Neurologist, 14*(5), 299–306.

Lally, R. (2014). Pesticide exposure linked to Alzheimer's disease. *Rutgers Today.* Retrieved from http://news.rutgers.edu/research-news/pesticide-exposure-linked-alzheimer%E2%80%99s-disease/20140127#.VCFcyhZP3-E

Mayo Clinic. (2014). Alzheimer's disease in-depth. Retrieved from http://www.mayoclinic.org/diseases-conditions/alzheimers-disease/in-depth/CON-20023871

Mayo Clinic. (2013). Lewy body dementia. Retrieved from http://www.mayoclinic.org/diseases-conditions/lewy-body-dementia/basics/definition/con-20025038

Mayo Clinic. (2014). Vascular dementia. Retrieved from http://www.mayoclinic.org/diseases-conditions/vascular-dementia/basics/definition/con-20029330

McKhann, G.M., Knopman, D.S., Chertkow, H., Hyman, B.T., Jack, C.R. Jr., Kawas, C.H., … & Phelps, C.H. (2011). The diagnosis of dementia due to Alzheimer's disease: Recommendations from the National Institute on Aging-Alzheimer's Association workgroups on diagnostic guidelines for Alzheimer's disease. *Alzheimer's and Dementia, 7*, 263–269.

National Institute of Mental Health. (n.d.). Signs and symptoms of depression. Retrieved from http://www.nimh.nih.gov/health/topics/depression/men-and-depression/signs-and-symptoms-of-depression/index.shtml

National Institute of Neurological Disorders and Stroke. (2015). Creutzfeldt-Jakob disease fact sheet. Retrieved from http://www.ninds.nih.gov/disorders/cjd/detail_cjd.htm

National Institute on Aging. (2015). Retrieved from http://www.nia.nih.gov/

NIH Senior Health. (n.d.). Alzheimer's disease. Retrieved from http://nihseniorhealth.gov/alzheimersdisease/symptomsanddiagnosis/01.html

Saunders, P. (2012). Alzheimer's vs. normal aging: Six ways to tell the difference. *Examiner.* Retrieved from http://www.examiner.com/article/is-it-alzheimer-s-disease-or-normal-aging-six-ways-to-tell-the-difference

Smith, M.A., Casadesus, G., Joseph, J.A., & Perry, G. (2002). Amyloid-beta and tau serve antioxidant functions in the aging and Alzheimer brain. *Free Radical Biology and Medicine, 33*(9), 1195–1199.

Thompson, S., Lanctot, K.L., & Herrmann, N. (2004). The benefits and risks associated with cholinesterase inhibitor therapy in Alzheimer's disease. *Expert Opinion on Drug Safety, 3*(5), 425-440.

Wegerer, J. (2014). The connection between UTIs and dementia. Retrieved from http://www.alzheimers.net/2014-04-03/connection-between-utis-and-dementia/

Wilkinson, D.G., Francis, P.T., Schwam, E., & Payne-Parrish, J. (2004). Cholinesterase inhibitors used in the treatment of Alzheimer's disease: The relationship between pharmacological effects and clinical efficacy. *Drugs and Aging, 21*(7), 453-478.

Made in the USA
San Bernardino, CA
07 November 2019